Legal & Disclaimer

The information contained in this book is not designed to replace or take the place of any form of medication or professional medical advice. The information in this book has been provided for educational and entertainment purposes only.

The information contained in this book has been compiled from sources deemed reliable, and it is accurate to the best of the Author's knowledge. However, the Author cannot guarantee its accuracy and validity so cannot be held liable for any errors or omissions. Changes are periodically made to this book. You must consult your doctor or get professional medical advice before using any of the suggested remedies, techniques, or information in this book.

Upon using the information contained in this book, you agree to hold harmless the Author from and against any damages, costs and expenses, including any legal fees, potentially resulting from the application of any of the information provided by this guide. This disclaimer applies to any damages or injury caused by the use and application, whether directly or indirectly, of any advice or information presented, whether for breach of contract, tort, negligence, personal injury, criminal intent, or under any other cause of action.

You agree to accept all the risks of using the information presented inside this book. You need to consult a professional medical practitioner in order to ensure you are both able & healthy enough to participate in this program.

Contents

Introduction

In almost all forms of diet, carbohydrates make up the bulk of a person's dietary needs. Even more so in a vegetarian diet, where wheat, vegetables, and fruits are the center of it. on the other hand, a ketogenic diet is just the opposite of that. This particular diet relies on fat and protein, and little or no carbohydrates at all. So why then, does the concept of Ketogenic Vegan diet exist? How can two seemingly conflicting diet plans marry well together? What are the benefits in adopting the keto-vegan diet?

This book aims not only to help readers understand the theories and basics behind the Keto-vegan diet, but to also provide a workable, realistic diet plan that they can base on. With the wealth of recipes included in this book - ranging from breakfast, lunch, dinner, and even to desserts – readers who are interested in adopting this lifestyle can take the crucial first small steps towards a healthier and cleaner lifestyle. And finding common ground between the Keto and a vegan diet isn't too complicated as one may think.

The Ketogenic Diet

You may have heard about the Keto diet – or maybe you haven't. Whatever the case, this diet has most recently been popularized and is now gaining traction worldwide. But the origins of Keto diet isn't too recent – in fact, it has been around since the 1920s. Back then, it was originally developed as a a successful way to manage and control epileptic symptoms such as seizures. To break it down, keto diet is one with an extremely low or no-carbohydrates at all, thus forcing the body into a state of ketosis, which is a mild form of ketoacidosis. In this state of ketosis, ketone bodies start to build up in the bloodstream. Ketone bodies are produced by the liver and used as sources of energy when glucose is not readily available. So by depriving the body of readily available sugar sources such as carbohydrates and glucose, the body turns to burning ketones instead. When it does, the body begins to burn out fat, leading to weight loss.

Nowadays, the keto diet isn't so much a treatment method for seizures anymore, with the advent of anti-convulsives. Instead, it has gained recent popularity among dieters who have experienced significant, rapid weight loss with only a few side effects. It also helps in managing fatigue associated with the intake of processed food, keeping the blood sugar levels stable and producing a more stable flow of energy.

However, the keto diet works best only for short-term. If you're planning to lose muscle weight – that's where the keto diet falls short. Most of the weight it's trimming down is water weight, and with prolonged, continued practice without proper supervision, it can do more harm than good. Instead of doing the keto diet for weight loss, people should be in it to keep food in perspective, to nourish themselves properly, and to stay well.

The Vegan Diet

People who have decided to take up a vegan lifestyle do so for a number of ethical, environmental, or health reasons. Veganism is simply defined as a way of living that excludes all forms of animal products, including meat, dairy, and eggs.

Among vegans, there are different varieties that include:

- **Whole-food vegan diet:** A diet based on a wide variety of whole plant foods such as fruits, vegetables, whole grains, legumes, nuts, and seeds.

- **Raw-food vegan diet:** A vegan diet based on raw fruits, vegetables, nuts, seeds, or plant foods cooked at temperatures below 118F.

- **80/10/10:** This is a type of raw food diet that limits fat-rich plants such as nuts and avocados and relies mainly on raw fruits and soft greens instead.

There are still a host of varieties of vegan diets, but since most scientific research rarely notes the differences between them, most vegan diets are referred to as one specific kind. In general, the vegan diet seems to be particularly effective at keeping blood sugar levels at bay, explained by the higher fiber intake, which may blunt the blood sugar response. Observational studies also show that vegans are at a lower risk of developing heart disease. On the other hand, poorly planned vegan diets can put you at risk for certain deficiencies. In order to meet the adequate requirements, one should develop a diet plan that is rich in nutrients and provides enough for the daily needs of the body.

Chapter 1 - The Keto-vegan Diet

The Theory Behind

Not that we've taken a look into the keto and vegan diet individually, it is time for us to understand how a keto-vegan diet works. Essentially, it is a regular ketogenic diet without disregarding vegan ethics. It is a diet that exploits every advantage of a keto diet and in turn improves your health, cuts down on the abuse and cruelty against animals, and reduces your carbon footprint.

So how exactly does it work? Severe restriction on the intake of carbs deprives your body of glucose, the primary source of fuel to the cells. The body then turns to burning up fat reserves which can provide a whole lot of health benefits. And it doesn't end there – the increased intake of fat and protein coupled with reduced carb intake can help ensure that you're getting all the nutrients you need with none of the added ingredients and chemicals that you don't. According to studies, a higher intake of fat and protien can help supress your appetite and ghrelin, recognized as the hunger hormone. And although it can be challenging to swap out meat products towards plant-based ones, it can be done.

Just like a standard keto diet, the key is to trade in starchy veggies for low-carb vegetarian options. Most regular keto plans emphasize the consumption of animal-based products such as grass-fed butter and unprocessed meats, which can be hard. Fortunately, there are plenty of high-fat, plant-based choices readily available.

Benefits and What to Expect

1.   Burn fat and maintain a healthy weight

For many dieters, the keto diet along is enough to produce a significant drop in their weight in such a short span of time. But if that isn't your main goal, you can still enjoy its benefits to a more sustained and weight loss, when used long term and under the supervision of a professional. You can easily manage your weight by adopting this low carb, high fat diet because as your body enters into a state of ketosis, it will continue to burn fat until it reaches a healthy weight. Even without intensive exercise, you will find that this diet forces the body to burn fat instead of carbohydrates for its energy.

2.   Have more energy and less hunger cravings

When you are on a diet high in carbs, your body is ins a constant state of converting carbs into glucose, thereby elevating blood sugar levels. This is especially true when you are consuming large amounts of simple carbohydrates such as processed foods and sugars. As a result of this initial spike of energy from carbs, you begin to feel a rapid decline which makes you feel craving for more carbs to bring your energy back up. With the keto diet however, burning fats take much longer, so you can have consistent energy levels without the energy spikes and without any of the carb cravings.

3.   Reduce symptoms of epilepsy

The keto diet is an established and effective therapy for forms of epilepsy that are either medicine-resistant or difficult to treat.

4.   Protect and nourish the brain

Being around for the past 90 years, this diet is widely recognized by medical professionals, and recent evidence have found that it can also be useful to prevent a host of neurodegenerative disorders such as Alzheimer's disease, Parkinsons, sleep disorders and other diseases.

5.   Reduce the risk of diabetes

Consuming carbs cause our blood sugar called glucose, to rise rapidly in the bloodstream. When there is a constant increase, it can lead to a whole host of problems such as insulin resistance and eventually obesity or type 2 diabetes. On the other hand, the ketogenic prevents this sugar spike because of the high consumption of fat. Many type 2 diabetics are also able to reduce or discontinue their medications after adopting the keto diet.

6.   Reduce the possibility of metabolic syndrome

Because the keto diet changes the way your body processes fats, it has been shown to actually reduce abdominal fat as well as triglycerides. Other benefits also include reduced blood sugar as well as decreased LDL and increased HDL.

Dealing with Side Effects

With the monumental swing that is happening to the popularity of the keto diet, a lot of attention is now focused on what makes it so effective and what to do when it doesn't deliver good on its promised effects. Considering that the goal of the keto diet is is to completely alter the way your body processes energy in order to burn fat, side effects come hardly as a surprise. And while not everyone gets to experience the same side effects, knowing how to take control and manage them can be very helpful.

One of the most prevalent side effects associated with the keto diet is known as "keto flu". While it's not really a flu, the symptoms are similar. It occurs because as the body enters ketosis, it increases the production of of urine and frequency of urination. This result to symptoms similar to dehydration, causing dizziness, nausea, headache, and irritability among others. Simply increasing your intake of salt and water can help relieve symptoms.

Another common side effect you may experience is an intense craving for sweets. Since the brain interprets a low blood sugar level in the body as starvation, it triggers an emergency signal that immediately makes you want to consume high sugar and high carb foods. Sugar craving swill and go, and the only way you can withstand them is to wait them out. Eventually, your body will get used to the new source of energy, and these cravings will soon disappear.

You may also start to feel a decrease in physical strength and overall performance as you're making the transition to the keto diet. note that is only temporary and is used as a period of learning where your body adapts to these changes and takes them on eventually. Once past this crucial period, your strength and energy will will return in an even greater capacity than ever.

Do's and Don'ts

If you're wondering where to get started and confused about how to get things rolling, here are some basic ground rules for following the keto-vegan diet:

- The keto-vegan diet should not include any meat or animal products, including dairy, eggs, and honey.

- The standard keto diet should be consisting of 75% calories from fat, 20% from protein, and just 5% from carbohydrates.

- Reduce your intake of high-carbs such as starchy veggies, sugary fruits, legumes, and grains.

- Stock up on low-carb and nutrient-rich foods such as nuts, seeds, low-carb fruits and veggies, leafy greens, healthy fats, and fermented foods.

- Make sure to restrict your carbs below 35g per day and stick to plenty of fat and protein consumption.

Being one of the most sustainable diets in the planet, the vegan keto diet can easily give desirable results. It is also worth noting that there are food sources that are more recommended than others, and that there are certain food you should limit or totally avoid. For best results, stick to these keto-vegan friendly foods.

Keto-vegan Friendly Foods	Examples
Vegan "meats"	Tempeh, seitan, other high-protein, low-carb "meats"
Leafy greens	Spinach, collard greens, swiss chard, kale
Vegetables that grow above ground	Broccoli, cauliflower, zucchini
Fat sources/ oil	Coconut oil, olive oil, MCT oil, and red palm oil, sesame oil, avocados
Low carb berries	Raspberries, blackberries, and strawberries
Vegan dairy	Coconut yogurt, almond milk, coconut milk, coconut cream, and vegan cheese

Nut butters	Almond butter, coconut butter, sunflower seed butter
Low carb sweeteners	Stevie and Erythritol

Likewise, these are the foods to avoid:

Foods To Avoid	**Examples**
Grains	Wheat, corn, rice, cereal
Legumes	Lentils, black beans, peas
Sugar Sources	Honey, agave, maple syrup
Fruits	Apples, bananas, oranges
Tubers	Potatoes, yam

Always try to be vigilant with what you eat. This is because most vegan staples like rice, quinoa, lentils, and beans are not allowed in the keto-vegan diet. It can definitely be quite challenging to restrict your net carbs while increasing your protein and fat intake. But with a little planning, it'll be a breeze in no time.

Food Substitutions

<u>Fat Sources</u>

Most plant-based oils are great options to replace every animal fat generally used in baking and cooking.

- Red Palm oil – Cooking with this enhances the flavors of your seeds, nuts, and vegan meat, giving it a rich and buttery taste. It is rich in vitamins A and E, acting as a natural supplement to your diet.

- Olive Oil – One of the healthiest cooking oils around, olive oil enhances the fat content and flavor of your meals. Make sure to keep it a temperature of less than 405F when cooking in order to preserve its health benefits.

- MCT Oil – This is a common derivative of palm oil and coconut oil. It can be added to your tea or coffee, as well as fat bombs, smoothies, salads dressings, and sauces.

- Coconut Oil – This is a great oil for baking and cooking at temperatures below 350F.

- Avocado Oil – With the highest smoking point of any other cooking oil at 520F, this oil is perfect for deep frying, baking, and cooking.

- Seeds – Seeds provide a healthy high fat addition to your meals. Examples include sunflower seeds, flaxseeds, sesame seeds, and pumpkin seeds.

- Nuts – Nuts such as cashews and macadamia have a high amount of mono-saturated fats as well as omega 6 fats.

- Avocado – This fruit is loaded with vitamins, minerals, and antioxidants. Make it a healthy addition to your meals and desserts.

Dairy Alternatives

There are healthy plant-based substitutes for cheese, yogurt, cream, and butter. Instead of eggs, one can use Vegg or VeganEgg. For sour cream and yogurt, there are nut-based yogurts in place. Vegan soft cheese can be used in place of cream cheese, while vegetarian cheese can replace dairy-based cheeses. Vegetarian butter or coconut oil can be used instead of butter and coconut cream in place of heavy cream.

Protein Sources

Seeds and nuts – Flaxseeds, sunflower seeds, almonds, pistachios, and pumpkin seeds are all great sources of protein but be careful with their consumption because they also contain carbs.

Seitan – Also known as wheat meat, it is a veggie replacement made from seaweed, garlic, ginger, soy sauce, and wheat gluten. It is a good source of iron, low in fat and high in protein.

Organic Tempeh – This fermented form of soy can replace ground meat and fish, and is more grainy and firmer than tofu.

Organic Tofu – Made from soybeans, tofu is high in calcium and protein, can be used to replace meat and fish in your meals.

Chapter 2 – Vegan Ketogenic Recipes

Breakfast Recipes

Ginger-baked Plums

Servings: 5

Prep Time: 10 minutes   Cook Time: 20 minutes

Ingredients:

2 pcs Ginger, peeled and grated

5 Plums, pitted and segmented into 8

Zest of 1 Orange

½ tsp Cinnamon

5 tbsp water

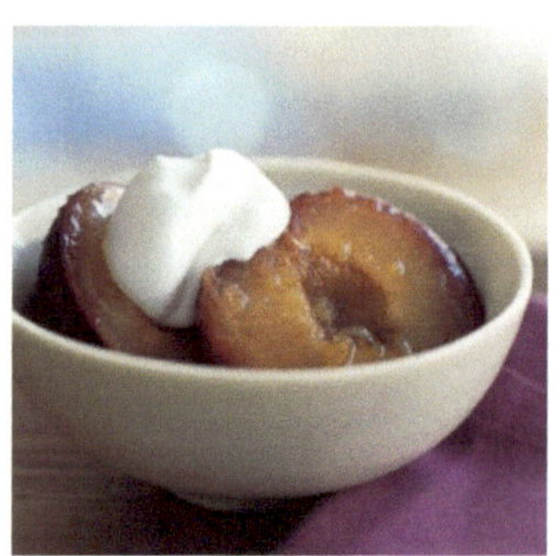

Procedure:

1.   Heat up an oven to 375F.

2.   Place the plums flesh side down on the baking tray.

3.   Mix together orange zest, grated ginger, water, and cinnamon in a bowl.

4.   Stir well and top over prepared plums.

5.   Bake for 20 minutes. Allow to cool.

6.   Serve topped with coconut yogurt if desired.

Walnut Porridge

Servings: 2

Prep Time: 10 minutes   Cook Time: 5 minutes

Ingredients:

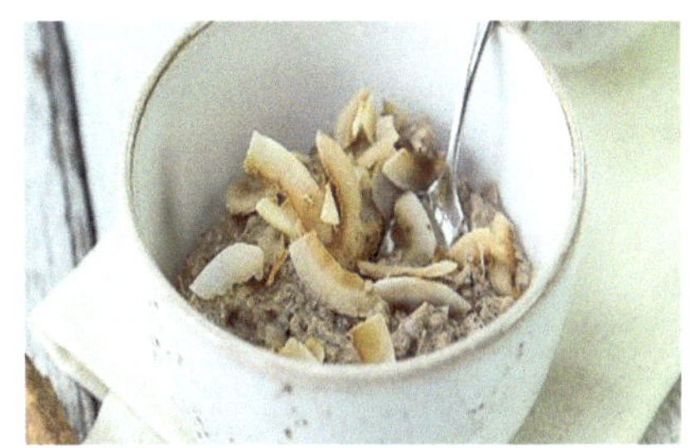

¼ cup coconut milk

¾ cup unsweetened almond milk

2 tbsp whole chia seeds

½ cup walnuts, chopped

2 tbsp hemp seeds

Procedure:

1. In a saucepan over medium heat, pour in almond milk, and coconut milk. Stir mixture until warm.

2. Remove the mixture from heat and stir in chopped walnuts, chia seeds, and hemp seeds.

3. Stir until combined and set aside for 5-10 minutes.

4. Scoop porridge into serving bowls and top with toasted coconut if desired.

5. Serve hot or cold.

Coconut Cream Berry Bowl

Servings: 4

Preparation Time: 15 minutes

Ingredients:

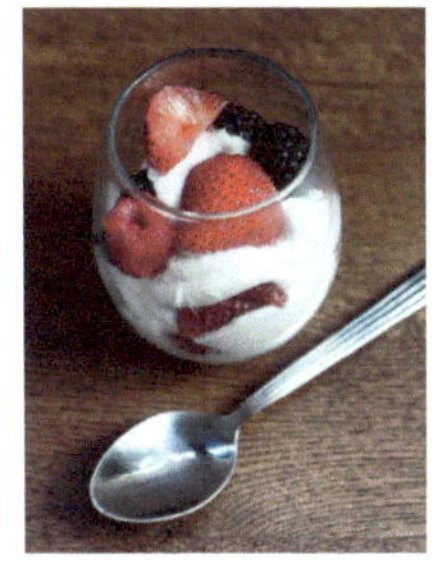

5 pcs fresh mint leaves, minced

4 cups of your desired fresh berries

1 whole vanilla pod

1 can full-fat coconut milk, chilled

1 tsp birch xylitol

Procedure:

1. Chop mixed berries into small chunks and place in a big mixing bowl.

2. Add the minced mint leaves into the bowl and toss until combined. Set aside.

3. Scoop out the solidified coconut milk from the container and into a bowl. Remove the coconut liquid.

4. Cut ends of vanilla pod and scrape the seeds. Add this to the bowl of coconut cream.

5. Beat vanilla seeds with coconut cream until well mixed.

6. Add birch xylitol into the mixture.

7. Continue mixing until a fluffy consistency is reached.

8. Top with berries and fresh mint leaves mixture.

Raspberry Chia Pudding

Servings: 2

Preparation Time: 15 minutes

Ingredients:

½ cup water

1 cup coconut milk

½ cup whole chia seeds

1 cup frozen or fresh raspberries

2-3 tsp unsweetened vanilla extract

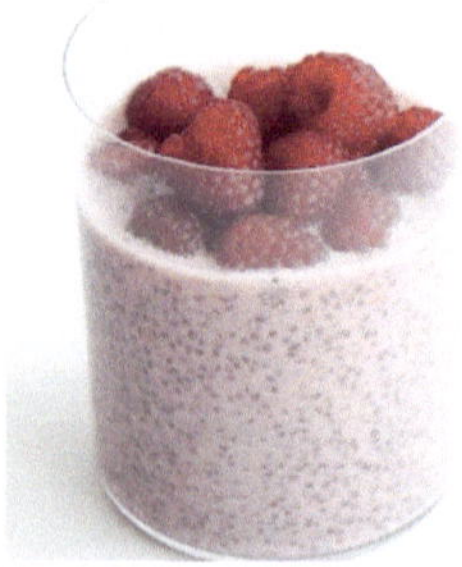

Procedure:

1. In a blender, add raspberries, water, and coconut milk.

2. Process until completely blended.

3. Combine Stevia (optional), vanilla, raspberry milk, and chia seeds in a mixing bowl and chill for 25-30 minutes.

4. Scoop into serving glasses and top with extra raspberries.

Bagel Thins

Servings: 4

Prep Time: 10 minutes   Cook Time: 40 minutes

Ingredients:

½ cup tahini

3 tbsp flaxseed, ground

½ cup psyllium husk powder

Pinch of salt

1 tsp baking powder

Sesame seeds for garnish

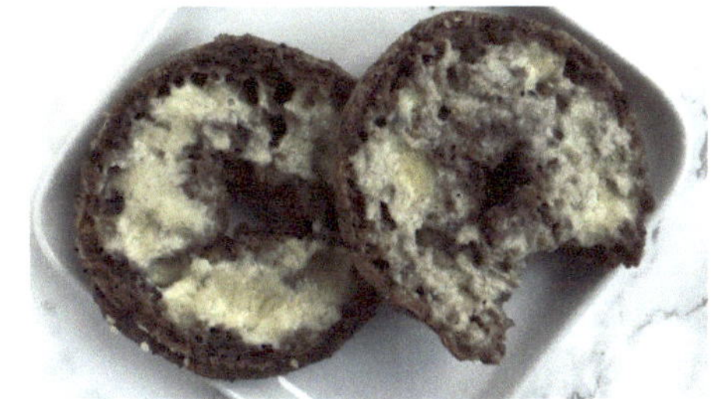

Procedure:

1. Heat oven to 375F.

2. Add salt, baking powder, ground flax seeds, and psyllium husk powder into a mixing bowl.

3. Whisk well to combine.

4. Add 1 cup water into this dry mixture and stir to combine until the water is absorbed.

5. Add the tahini and stir until dough is incorporated, even, and consistent.

6. Shape the batter into ¼ inches thick patties.

7. Arrange patties on a baking tray and poke a small circle in the center of each patty.

8. Top with sesame seeds and transfer to preheated oven. Bake for about 40 minutes, until golden brown.

9. Cut into 2 and toast as you would with a regular bagel. Serve with your desired toppings or spreads.

Hemp Heart Porridge

Servings: 1

Prep Time: 2 minutes   Cook Time: 3 minutes

Ingredients:

1 cup vegan (almond or coconut) milk

2 tbsp flax seeds, freshly ground

½ cup hemp hearts

1 tbsp chia seeds

½ tsp cinnamon, ground

¾ tsp pure vanilla extract

¼ cup ground almonds

Hemp hearts and Brazil nuts for toppings

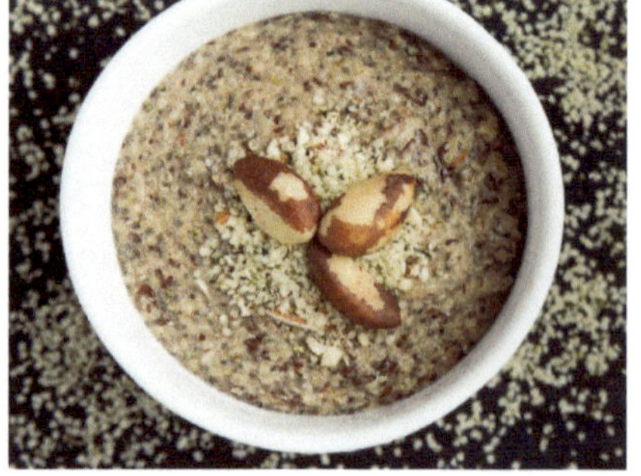

Procedure:

1. Mix together all ingredients except the toppings and ground almonds into a small saucepan over medium heat.

2. Stir to combine.

3. Cook until just mixture boils slightly. Stir.

4. Turn off the heat and add crushed almonds.

5. Stir until combined and pour into bowl.

6. Add hemp seeds and Brazil nuts. Serve.

Vegan Protein Shake

Servings: 1

Prep Time: 5 minutes

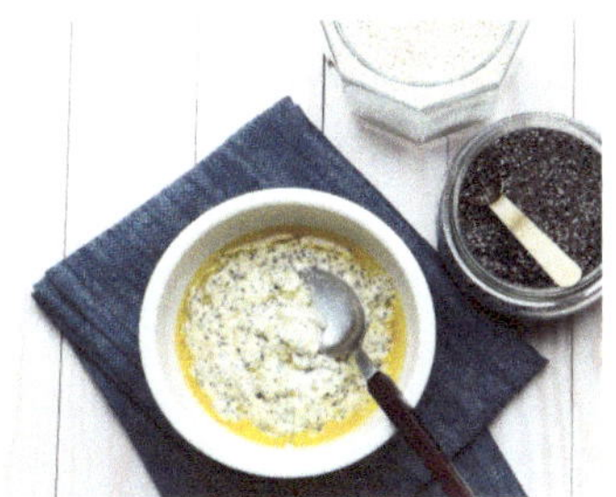

Ingredients:

2/3 cup full fat coconut milk

1 tbsp chia seed

½ cup hemp hearts

½ tsp vanilla extract

Pinch of Himalayan rock salt

Procedure:

1.   Add all ingredients together into a container with a lid and cap of securely.

2.   Stir well until combined.

3.   Refrigerate this covered container in the chiller overnight.

4.   Take out the container and add milk to desired thinness or thickness.

5.   Sprinkle with your favorite toppings and enjoy.

Flaxseed Waffles

Servings: 2

Prep Time: 10 minutes   Cook Time: 15 minutes

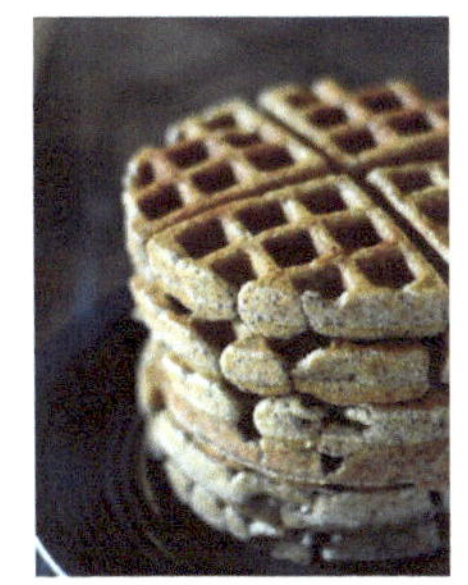

Ingredients:

2 cups golden flaxseed, coarsely ground

1 tbsp baking powder, gluten-free

5 flax eggs (5 tbsp flax meal + 12 tbsp hot water)

1 tbsp fresh herbs or 2 tsps ground cinnamon

1/3 cup melted coconut oil or avocado oil

Procedure:

1. Set waffle maker to desired heat setting.

2. Prepare the flax eggs by combining flax meal to hot water and set aside.

3. Add a pinch of sea salt, baking powder, and flax seed into a big mixing bowl.

4. Whisk until completely combined and let sit.

5. Add oil, ½ cup water, and flax eggs into a blender and blend until combined.

6. Transfer this into a bowl and and stir until fluffy.

7. Fold in fresh herbs or cinnamon.

8. Scoop a portion of the batter and pour into heated waffle machine.

9. Cook until done and serve.

Tofu Veggie Scramble

Servings: 2

Prep Time: 5 minutes   Cook Time: 10 minutes

Ingredients:

3 tbsp olive oil

3 tomatoes, chopped

4 garlic cloves, minced

1 cup fresh mushrooms, sliced

10 bunches fresh spinach

2 pounds firm tofu

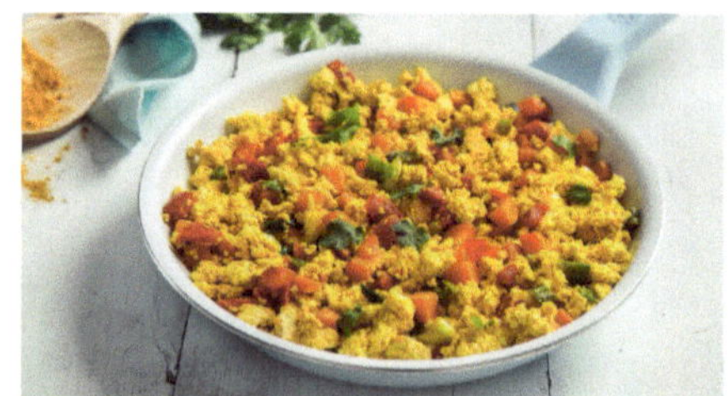

Procedure:

1. In a skillet, heat olive oil.

2. Saute tomatoes, garlic, and mushrooms for 2-3 minutes.

3. Reduce heat to medium-low and add spinach, crumbled tofu, and to taste, some soy sauce and lemon juice.

4. Cover and cook for another 5-7 minutes. Stir occasionally.

5. Sprinkle with salt and pepper. Serve.

Eggplant Hole

Servings: 2

Prep Time: 10 minutes   Cook Time: 20 minutes

Ingredients:

1 whole eggplant

1 tbsp extra virgin olive oil

1 tsp salted butter

4 whole pasteurized eggs

2 stalks green onions

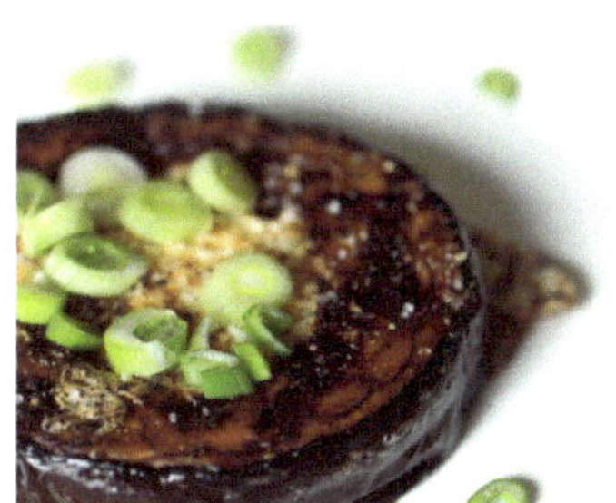

Procedure:

1. Preheat grill to high heat.

2. Rinse the eggplant then cut into1-inch slices.

3. Brush eggplant with olive oil and sprinkle with salt and pepper.

4. Grill eggplant on each side for about 3-4 minutes each.

5. Cut a hole in the center of each eggplant using a small cookie cutter.

6. Saute eggplants in a heated pan. Pour egg mixture into the center of each eggplant.

7. Allow egg to cook. Serve topped with sliced green onions as garnish.

Lunch and Dinner Recipes

Spicy Vegan Soup

Servings: 2

Prep Time: 10 minutes   Cook Time: 20 minutes

Ingredients:

2 tsp yellow mustard seed

2 cup green cabbage, minced

¼ tsp turmeric, ground

2 small red and green each, bell pepper, minced

2 medium yellow onion, minced

1 pc Habanero pepper, minced

4 cups water

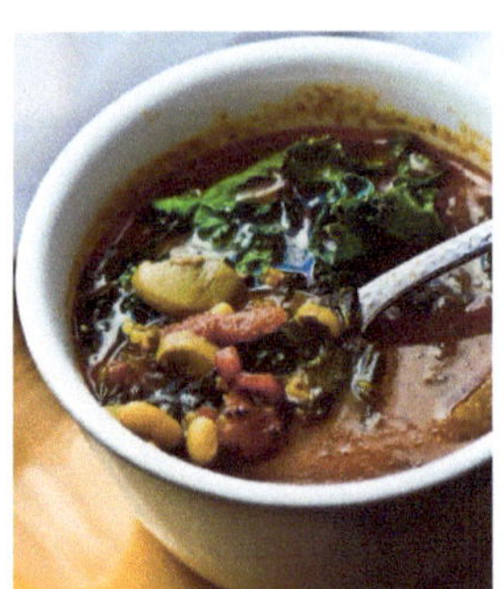

Procedure:

1.   Stir together 4 cups water, and spices in a pot.

2.   Add the vegetables over medium heat.

3.   Simmer until the mixture has a syrupy consistency and veggies are broken down.

4.   Serve warm.

Tomato-based Spaghetti Squash

Servings: 1-2

Prep Time: 15 minutes   Cook Time: 50 minutes

Ingredients:

½ tbsp olive oil or coconut oil

1 large spaghetti squash, halved width-wise or length-wise and seeded

1 can of Tomato sauce

2 cups of mixed bell peppers

2 cups of broccoli

Salt, as needed

Optional: vegan cheese

Procedure:

1.   Heat oven to 400F.

2.   Pour oil over halved spaghetti squash. Sprinkle salt as needed.

3.   Cover with aluminum foil to prevent burning at the top.

4.   Bake in the oven for 30 minutes.

5.   Cook bell peppers and broccoli in tomato sauce over medium heat.

6.   Take foil off spaghetti squash and bake for another 20 minutes.

7.   Once done, transfer to a cooling rack and rest for 10 minutes.

8.   Scrape out spaghetti strings from the squash with a fork..

9.   Mix spaghetti with tomato sauce mixture. Top with vegan cheese if desired.

Spinach – Artichoke Casserole

Servings: 5

Prep Time: 15 minutes   Cook Time: 3 hours

Ingredients:

8 flax eggs (8 tbsp flax meal plus 24 tbsp hot water)

5 ounces fresh spinach, chopped

¾ cup almond milk, unsweetened

1 cup vegan parmesan, grated or nutritional yeast

6 ounces chopped artichoke hearts

¾ cup coconut flour

Pepper, salt, minced garlic as needed

Optional: fresh basil

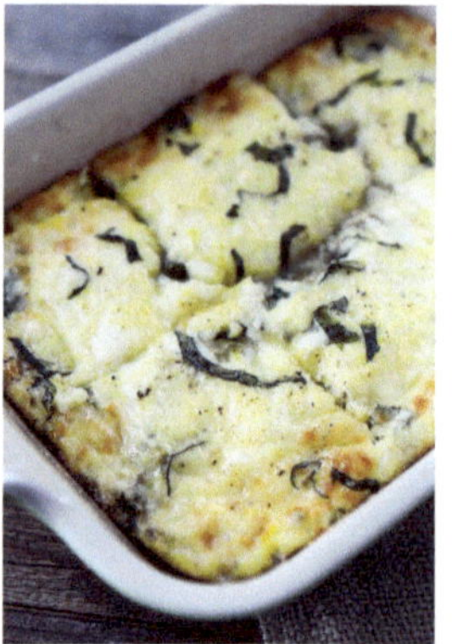

Procedure:

1.   Combine 8 tbsp flax meal with 24 tbsp hot water and set aside.

2.   Add pepper, salt, minced garlic, ½ cup grated parmesan or nutritional yeast, artichoke hearts, spinach, almond milk, and the flax eggs into a big bowl.

3.   Whisk thoroughly. Add in baking powder and coconut flour.

4.   Whisk until incorporated.

5.   Spread the flour mixture into a greased crock pot and sprinkle the reserved ½ cup parmesan on top.

6.   Cover and cook for 4-6 hours on low or 2-3 hours on high.

7.   Top with fresh basil and serve.

Stuffed Mushrooms

Servings: 3

Prep Time: 10 minutes   Cook Time: 22 minutes

Ingredients:

12 whole fresh mushrooms, caps intact, stems chopped finely

1 tbps garlic, minced

8 ounces vegan cream cheese

¼ tsp cayenne pepper, ground

2 tbsp vegan soy bacon bits

¼ tsp onion powder

¼ tsp pepper

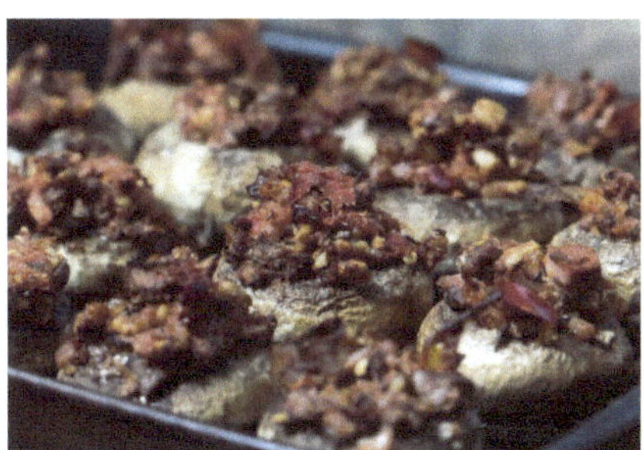

Procedure:

1. Heat oven to 350F. Prepare a greased baking pan.

2. Add vegetable oil into a skillet over medium heat.

3. Add mushroom stems and garlic into the hot oil and saute for 2 minutes.

4. Set aside and cool.

5. Combine vegan soy bacon bits, cayenne pepper, onion powder, pepper, vegan cream cheese, and cooled mushroom stems into a bowl.

6. Stir thoroughly until well blended.

7. Top each mushroom cap with the filling.

8. Transfer the caps on to the baking tray and bake for 20 minutes.

Mexican Cauliflower Rice

Servings: 4

Prep Time: 10 minutes   Cook Time: 15 minutes

Ingredients:

½ medium onion, diced

2 tbsp olive oil

1 tbsp chili powder

1 garlic clove, minced

1 pound cauliflower, riced

1 tsp cumin

1 can tomatoes, diced, no salt added

Toppings: cilantro, limes, sour cream, avocado, olive oil, jalapeno

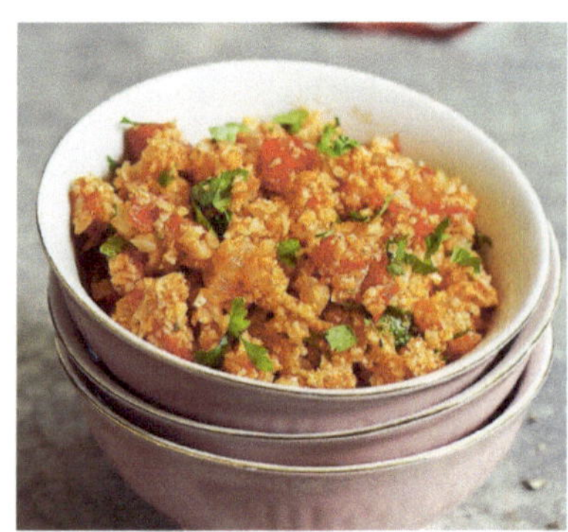

Procedure:

1.   In a pan, heat oil over medium heat.

2.   Add garlic and onion and cook for 2-3 minutes.

3.   Add spices into the mixture and cook until fragrant.

4.   Add the cauliflower rice and cook until crisp to the edges and tenderized.

5.   Add tomatoes into the skillet and stir until incorporated.

6.   Cook until rice has a fluffy consistency and dry, about 3-5 minutes more.

7.   Sprinkle salt as desired.

8.   Serve immediately.

Zucchini Noodles

Servings: 4

Prep Time: 10 minutes   Cook Time: 15 minutes

Ingredients:

½ cup avocado pesto

4 medium zucchinis, spiralized using a veggie spiralizer

1 cup kalamata olives, pitted

2 avocados, peeled, and sliced into thin strips

¼ cup drained sun-dried tomatoes

2 tbsp coconut oil

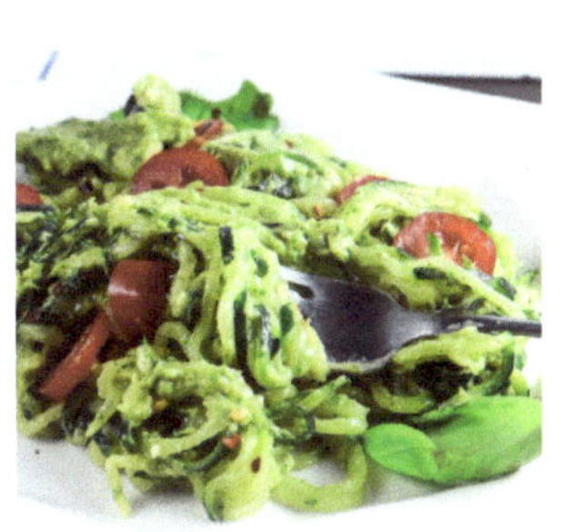

Procedure:

1. Chop the soft core of the zucchini and place in the bowl with the spiralized zucchini.

2. Transfer the zucchini noodles into a pan with coconut oil over medium heat.

3. Cook until desired softness, about 2-3 minutes.

4. Transfer cooked noodles into a bowl and add the pesto.

5. Top with fresh basil, olives, avocado and tomatoes.

Bibimbap

Servings: 2

Prep Time: 15 minutes   Cook Time: 10 minutes

Ingredients:

7 ounces tempeh, sliced into squares

4-6 broccoli florets, sliced into spears

1 small red bell pepper, julliened

½ cucumber, julliened

1 carrot, grated

2 tbsp sirracha or gochujang sauce

10 ounces riced cauliflower, raw

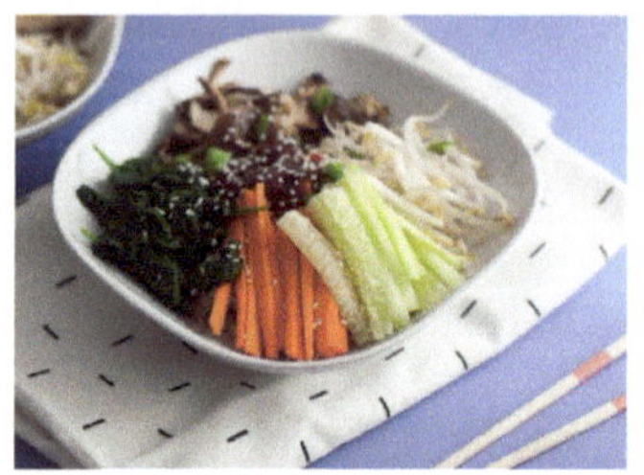

Procedure:

1. In a bowl, mix 1 tbsp soy sauce and vinegar until combined.

2. Immerse tempeh squares into the bowl and soak for 1-2 minutes.

3. Heat oil in a skillet over medium heat.

4. Fry soaked tempeh. Remove when brown and set aside.

5. Saute carrots, broccoli, and peppers until cooked. Set aside.

6. In another pan, heat oil and toss in riced cauliflower and cook until softened.

7. Add soy sauce and chili paste.

8. Portion the riced cauliflower into bowls. Add raw cucumber, the sauteed vegetables, and tempeh.

9. Top with chili sauce and sprinkle with sesame seeds.

Noodle Bowls in Curry Sauce

Servings: 2

Prep Time: 10 minutes   Cook Time: 15 minutes

Ingredients:

16 gm kanten noodles

2 carrots, julienned

½ head cauliflower, chopped

1 red bell pepper, diced

Handful fresh cilantro, chopped

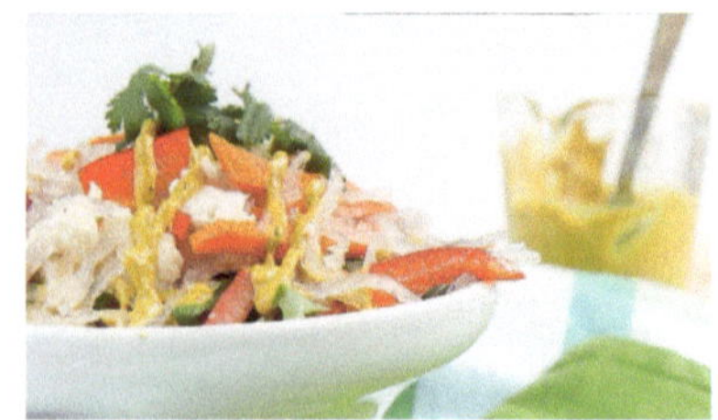

2 handfuls mixed greens

2 tbsp, Vegan curry sauce

Procedure:

1. Place 2 sheets of Kanten noodles in a bowl. Pour lukewarm water over to soak.

2. Add carrots, cauliflower, bell pepper, and cilantro to the bowl with noodles.

3. Set mixed greens on 2 plates to serve as your "base".

4. Pour ready mix curry sauce over vegetable noodle mix and serve.

Keto –Vegan Caesar Salad

Servings: 1

Prep Time: 5 minutes   Cook Time: 5 minutes

Ingredients:

1 ripe avocado

3 tbsp lemon juice

3 cloves garlic, minced

1 tbsp capers

2 tsps Dijon mustard

¼ cup hemp seeds

12 cups Romaine leaves, chopped

10 cherry tomatoes, halved

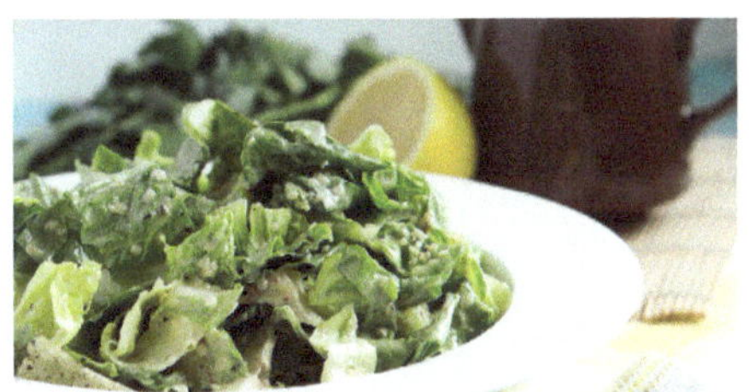

Procedure:

1. Add avocado, lemon juice, water, garlic, brine, capers, mustard, salt, and pepper to the bowl of your food processor or blender. Blend until smooth.

2. Spoon dressing into a bowl with hemp seeds and mix.

3. Place romaine and tomatoes in a large salad bowl and pour dressing on top.

Cream of Mushroom Soup

Servings: 2

Prep Time: 10 minutes   Cook Time: 30 minutes

Ingredients:

2 cups cauliflower florets

1 2/3 cup unsweetened original almond milk

1 tsp onion powder

½ tsp extra virgin olive oil

1 ½ cups mushrooms, diced

½ yellow onion, diced

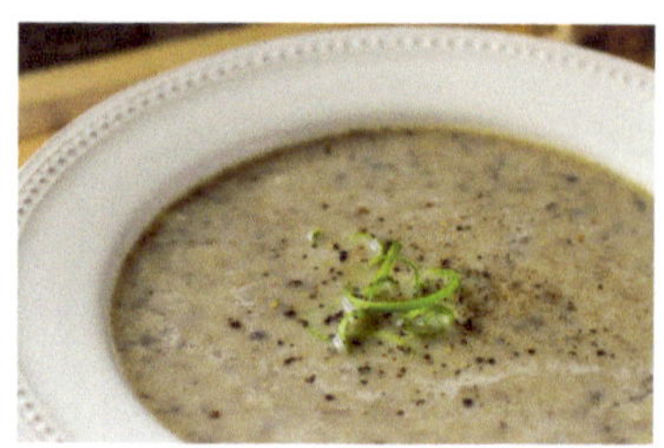

Procedure:

1. Place cauliflower, milk, onion powder, salt, and pepper in a saucepan. Bring to a boil over medium heat.

2. Reduce heat and simmer for 7-8 minutes until cauliflower is softened.

3. Puree this using an immersion blender or transfer to a blender.

4. In another pan, saute mushrooms and onions in oil. Continue cooking until onions are translucent.

5. Add pureed cauliflower mix to sauteed mushrooms. Bring to a boil, cover and simmer for 10 minutes until thickened.

6. Serve immediately.

Zucchini Lasagna with Walnut Tofu Sauce

Servings: 2

Prep Time: 10 minutes   Cook Time: 35 minutes

Ingredients:

1 cup walnuts, finely ground

25 ounces marinara sauce, divided

¼ cup sun-dried tomatoes, chopped

Lasagna:

2 zucchini

2 tbsp nutritional yeast, optional

14 oz firm tofu

1 tbsp lemon juice

salt and pepper

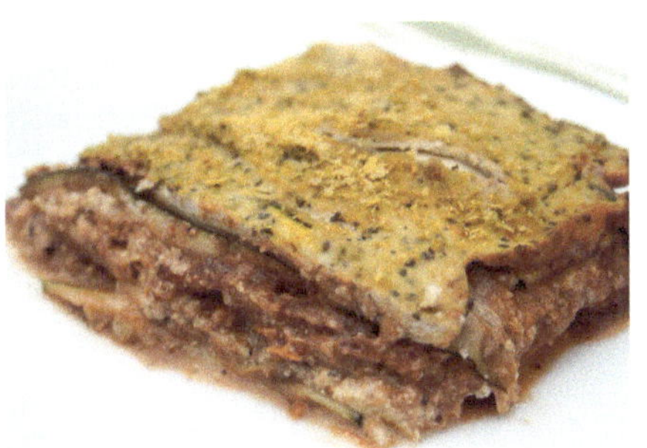

Procedure:

1. Mix together tofu, lemon juice, and olive oil in a food processor until smooth. Set aside.

2. Preheat oven to 375F.

3. Mix walnuts, marinara sauce, (reserve ¾ for the pan), and sun-dried tomatoes.

4. Slice zucchini 1/16 inches lengthwise on a mandolin.

5. In a 8x9inch pan, pour marinara sauce. Place zucchini noodles on marinara sauce, overlapping each slice. Spread 1/3 of tofu over zucchini noodles. Sprinkle nutritional yeast on top of tofu.

6. Pour half of walnut sauce on top.

7. Layer more zucchini noodles, then 1/3 of tofu, nutritional yeast, and the rest of the walnut sauce. Finish with another layer of zucchini topped with the remaining sauces.

8. Bake at 375F for 35 minutes.

Hemp Seed Cauliflower Pilaf

Servings: 1

Prep Time: 5 minutes   Cook Time: 5 minutes

Ingredients:

½ head of cauliflower

½ cup hemp seeds

4 pitted dates, chopped

½ tsp turmeric

½ tsp cumin

½ low sodium vegetable broth

¼ cup sliced almonds

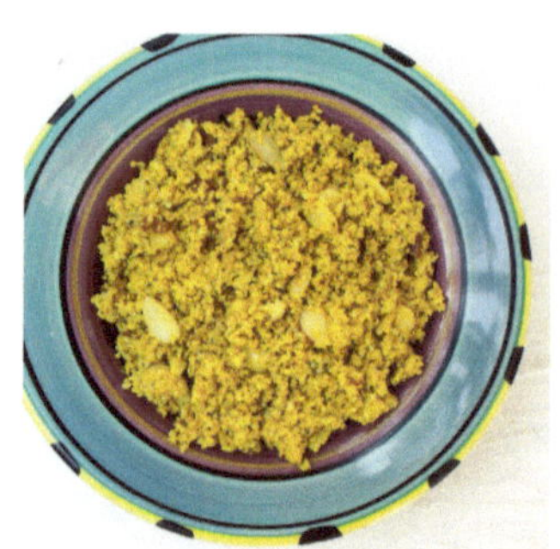

Procedure:

1. Place head of cauliflower in a food processor and mix until it resembles a rice consistency.

2. Place cauliflower rice in a pan along with hemp seeds, chopped dates, turmeric, cumin, vegetable broth, and salt and pepper.

3. Cook until liquid is absorbed, for about 5 minutes.

4. Add sliced almonds.

5. Serve immediately.

Ginger- Sesame Walnuts and Hemp seed Lettuce Wraps

Servings: 2

Prep Time: 10 minutes   Cook Time: 10 minutes

Ingredients:

1 cup walnuts, chopped

1 cup hemp seeds

4 dates, chopped

1 cup cucumber, chopped

½ cup carrots, chopped

Lettuce leaves

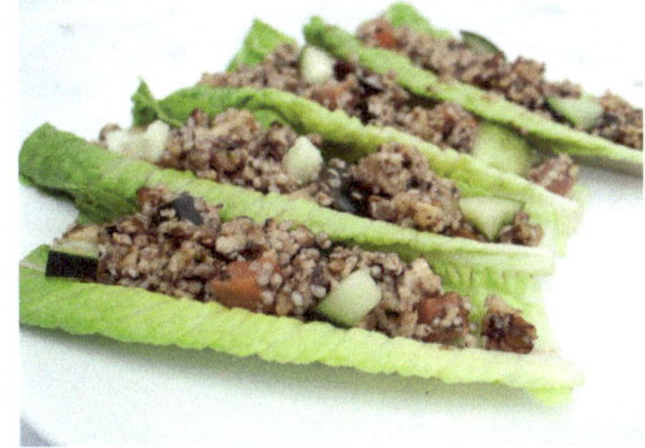

Sauce:

1 tbsp maple syrup

1 tsp roasted sesame oil

2 tbsp brown rice vinegar

1 tbsp minced ginger

Procedure:

1. Mix sauce ingredients.

2. Add in walnuts, hemp seeds, dates, cucumber, and carrots. Rest for about an hour in the fridge.

3. Pile mixture into lettuce leaves. Top with sesame seeds if desired.

Tempeh Stir-fry

Servings: 2

Prep Time: 10 minutes   Cook Time: 15 minutes

Ingredients:

8 ounces gluten-free tempeh cut into 1x2 inch rectangular strips

3 tbsps olive oil, divided

8 ounces shitake or button mushrooms halved and thinly sliced

8 ounces regular broccoli, cut into 2-inch segments

1 tbsp each ginger and garlic, minced

Dressing:

3 tbsp tahini

1 tbsp chili garlic sauce

2 tbsp tamari

1 tbsp sesame oil

1 tbsp maple syrup

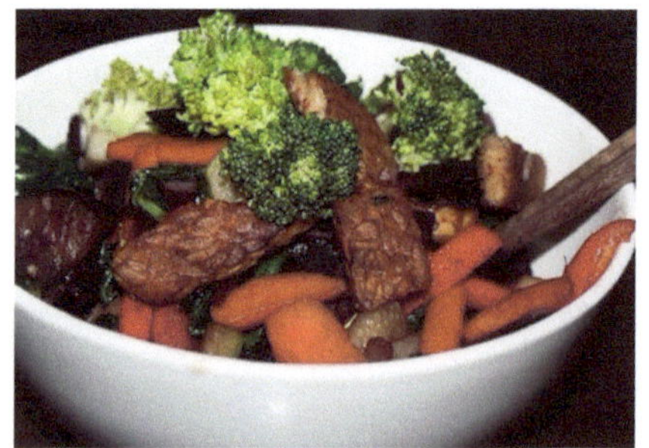

Procedure:

1.   Heat 2 tbsp oil over medium high-heat.

2.   Cook tempeh until browned. Set aside.

3.   To the same pan, add 1 tbsp oil and mushroom, and cook for a few minutes. Set aside.

4.   To the pan , add broccoli, ginger, and garlic. Cook for a few minutes.

5.   Add mushrooms and tempeh to pan and mix.

6.   In a small bowl, mix all sauce ingredients until smooth.

7.   Serve tempeh stir-fry drizzled with the sauce and serve immediately.

Jackfruit and Cauliflower Taco Bowls

Servings: 2

Prep Time: 5 minutes   Cook Time: 10 minutes

Ingredients:

1 can young jackfruit in water, drained

2 tbsp taco seasoning

1 cup kale, frozen

2 package cauliflower rice

1 tbsp olive oil

Vegan cheese and guacamole for serving

Procedure:

1. Chop jackfruit into smaller sizes.

2. Add everything in a pot except for the vegan cheese and guacamole. Saute until cauliflower is tender.

3. Serve with vegan cheese and guacamole.

Dessert Recipes

Chocolate and Orange Chia Pudding

Servings: 4

Preparation Time: 15 minutes

Ingredients:

1 cup coconut milk

½ cup chia seeds, ground or whole

2 tsp fresh orange zest

2 cup almond milk or water

15-20 drops orange Stevia extract

225g 85% dark chocolate

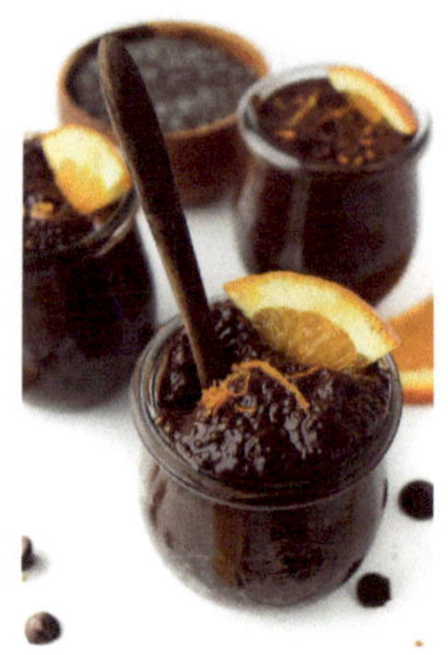

Procedure:

1. Add stevia as desired, fresh orange zest, almond milk or water, coconut milk, and chia seeds in a bowl.

2. Stir until combined.

3. Set mixture aside for 10-15 minutes or more.

4. Add grated dark chocolate. Stir until well combined.

5. Optional: top with coconut cream and serve.

Keto-vegan Granola

Servings: 10 - 14

Prep Time: 10 minutes   Cook Time: 50 minutes

Ingredients:

1 ¼ cup whole almonds

¼ cup pine nuts, pecans, and cashew nuts

½ cup sunflower seeds

1 cup unsweetened coconut, shaved or shredded

½ cup flax meal

½ cup coconut oil

¼ tsp each of cardamom and cinnamon

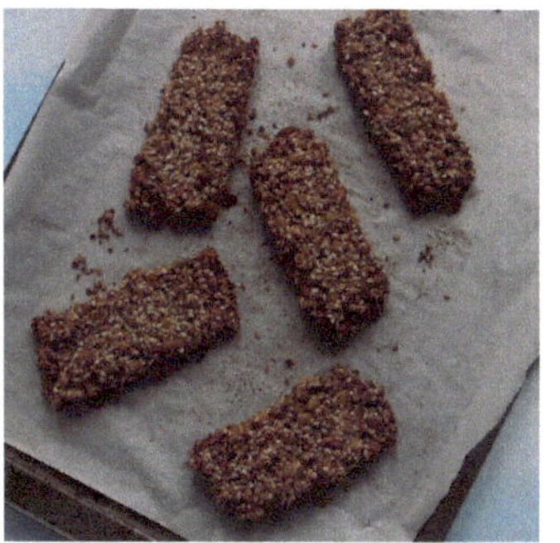

Procedure:

1. Heat oven to 300F.

2. Add all the spices, seeds, and nuts into a bowl and stir well until combined.

3. Add coconut oil into a pan and heat until melted.

4. Pour melted coconut oil into nut and seed mixture and mix until well combined.

5. Evenly spread nuts and seeds mixture on a parchment paper lined with baking tray.

6. Transfer this tray into the oven and bake for an hour. Stir once very 15 minutes, careful not to burn the mixture.

7. Once crunchy and browned, remove from oven.

8. If desired, sprinkle orange zest and sea salt. Allow to cool.

9. Once completely cooled, store well inside a container for up to 30 days.

10. Optional: Serve with coconut milk, cashew milk, or coconut yogurt.

Chocolate Pumpkin Mousse Pie

Servings: 10 - 12

Prep Time: 20 minutes   Cook Time: 15 minutes

Ingredients:

2 tbsp coconut oil, ¼ cup coconut oil

100gm 85% chocolate

1.2 cup coconut butter

2 tsp pumpkin spice mix

½ cup pumpkin puree, unsweetened

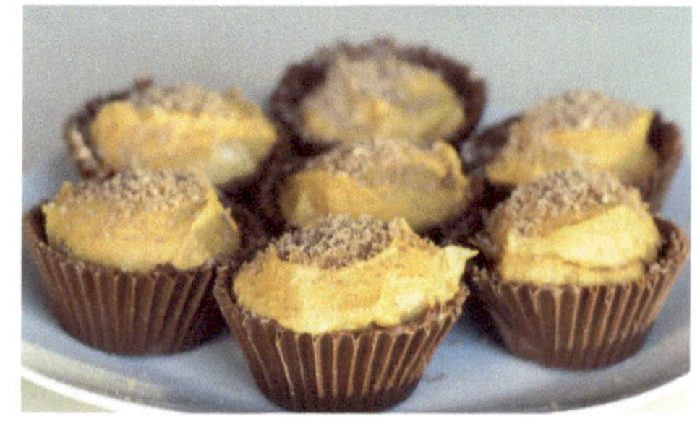

Procedure:

1. Add 2 tbsp coconut oil and chocolate into a double boiler over medium heat and melt the mixture.

2. Take the chocolate oil mixture off the heat and let it sit.

3. Scoop 2 tsp chocolate oil into 10 - 12 mini muffin cups.

4. Transfer to a chiller and cool for 10 minutes or more.

5. Add pumpkin spice mix, ¼ cup coconut oil, and coconut butter into a double boiler and melt.

6. To this, add the pumpkin puree.

7. Take out refrigerated cups and add a generous teaspoon of the coconut/pumpkin mixture into each cup.

8. Refrigerate for 30 minutes or more. Can be chilled up to 7 days and frozen for up to 90 days.

Chocolate Ice Cream

Servings: 2

Prep Time: 10 minutes

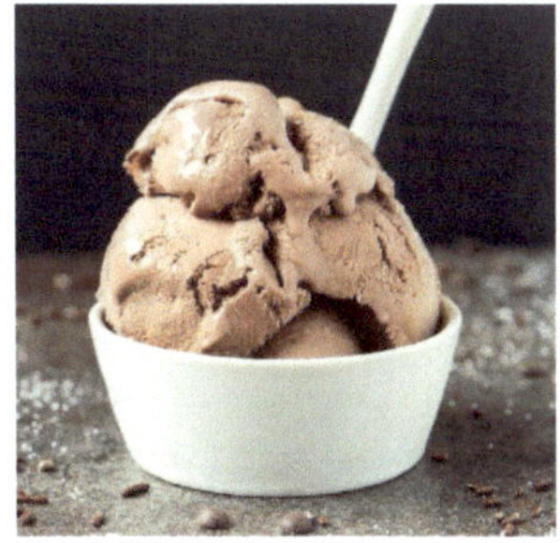

Ingredients:

½ cup + 1 tbsp 100% pure chocolate

1 can chilled coconut milk or very cold coconut milk

6 drops chocolate Stevia

¼ tsp clear Stevia drops, as necessary

Procedure:

1. Add all ingredients into a bowl.

2. Using an electric mixer, mix until smooth, thick, and frothy.

3. Add this mixture into a an ice cream maker and follow manufacturer's instructions.

4. Consume immediately. Otherwise, freeze until solidified and thaw for 20 minutes before eating.

Spiced Coconut Bars

Servings: 10

Prep Time: 10 minutes   Cook Time: 12 minutes

Ingredients:

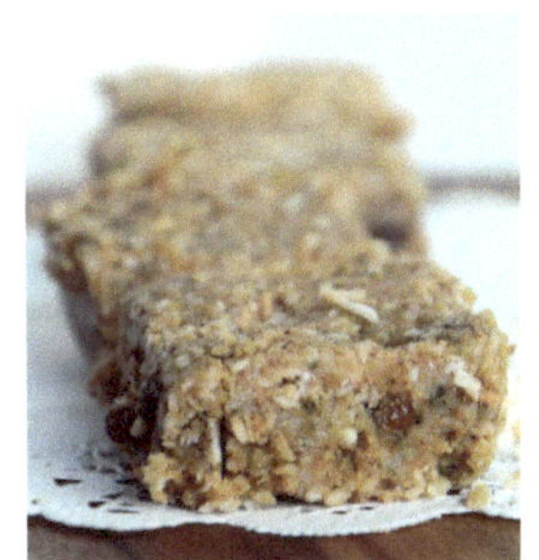

1 ¾ cup unsweetened coconut, shredded

3.5 ounces vegan butter or coconut oil

1½ cup coconut milk, unsweetened

1 tsp cardamom powder

10-20 saffron threads

Procedure:

1. Add 1 ¼ cup coconut milk and shredded coconut into a bowl.

2. Stir until combined and set aside for 30 minutes.

3. Add the saffron threads and remaining coconut milk into a bowl. Stir until well combined.

4. Melt coconut oil or vegan butter on a pan over medium heat.

5. To this, add the coconut mixture.

6. Cook for 5-7 minutes.

7. Add the cardamom powder and continue cooking for another 5 minutes. On a greased baking tray, spread the coconut mixture up to 1 cm thick.

8. Transfer into a freezer for 2 hours or more.

9. Cut coconut bars into squares and serve immediately.

Conclusion

Now that you're equipped with the theories and several recipes to start you on your journey, you are now ready to take that first step towards the Keto –vegan lifestyle. You may choose to stay on this diet for some time, or for a long time. Whichever the case may be, when you choose to do the keto-vegan diet, you will realize that as intimidating as it may seem at first, this is one hundred percent doable. Yes, the restrictions may be constricting at first, and your body will require a period of transition in which it will need to get used to the new regimen and the state of ketosis, but then again what kind of transition doesn't deal with changes?

The Keto –vegan diet satisfies all the necessary markers for a life of health – the natural reduction of calories, blood sugar control, boosted saturated fats, and a whole lot more. I hope that this book will serve as a safe and healthy jumping point for you.

Margaret Lane